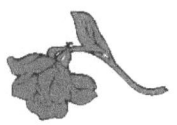

THE POWER OF THREE

By

Rose-marie Sinclair

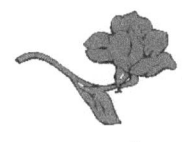

© Copyright 2009, Rose-marie Sinclair
www.alchemyrose.com
Email: alchemyrose@hotmail.com

All Rights Reserved.

No part of this book may be reproduced, stored in a
retrieval system, or transmitted by any means,
electronic, mechanical, photocopying, recording,
or otherwise, without written permission
from the author.

ISBN: 978-0-9757071-0-4

INTRODUCTION:

As a keeper of the Knowledge
The Moons of the Past
And the Suns of the Now
I Write from my Heart
And Think from my Brow
I know Love in Goodness
And Show Gratitude for All-That-Is.

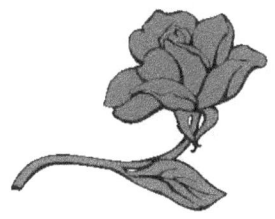

MISSION STATEMENT:

The Practitioner of the Now
Will Give Advice to Interest their Clients
In the Balance of the Human Frame,
In Energy Well-Being and
The Maintenance of Holistic Health.

HAPPINESS

Sun, sun glorious sun
Nothing quite like it
For having such fun.

Breath, breath glorious breath
Nothing quite like it
To keep us alive.

Love, love glorious love
Nothing quite like it
For moving the blood.

Sex, sex glorious sex
Nothing quite like it
To balance our lives.

Life, life glorious life
Nothing quite like it
To furnish our souls.

Earth, earth glorious earth
Nothing quite like it
For death and re-birth.

Water, water glorious water
Nothing quite like it
To recharge our cells.

Moon, moon glorious moon
Nothing quite like it
To flow with our dreams.

Time, time glorious time
Nothing quite like it
To live in the now.

Money, money glorious money
Nothing quite like it
To increase our bounty.

Beauty, beauty glorious beauty
Nothing quite like it
To know we are wealthy.

Joy, joy glorious joy
Nothing quite like it
To en-rich our thoughts

Peace, peace glorious peace
Nothing quite like it
To soothe heart and soul.

Passion, passion glorious passion
Nothing quite like it
To feel we're in heaven..

Choice, choice glorious choice
Nothing quite like it
To laugh and re-joice.

Freedom, freedom glorious freedom
Nothing quite like it
To excite our future.

THE POWER OF THREE

MESSAGE ONE:	CREATION	7
MESSAGE TWO:	TRINITY	10
MESSAGE THREE:	THE THIRD EYE	14
MESSAGE FOUR:	HERITAGE	17
MESSAGE FIVE:	ATTITUDE	20
MESSAGE SIX:	RESPONSIBILITY	23
MESSAGE SEVEN:	DIVINE WISDOM	26
MESSAGE EIGHT:	BALANCE	30
MESSAGE NINE:	PATIENCE	34
MESSAGE TEN:	CHARACTER	38
MESSAGE ELEVEN:	RELAXATION	41
MESSAGE TWELVE:	CREATIVITY	45
MESSAGE THIRTEEN:	CO-OPERATION	49
MESSAGE FOURTEEN:	PAIN	52
MESSAGE FIFTEEN:	FUN	55
MESSAGE SIXTEEN:	BEAUTY	57
MESSAGE SEVENTEEN:	ADVENTURE	60
MESSAGE EIGHTEEN:	FRIENDS AND FAMILY	63
MESSAGE NINETEEN:	PRIDE	67
MESSAGE TWENTY:	DIMENSIONAL SHIFT	70
MESSAGE TWENTY-ONE:	GRATITUDE	73
MESSAGE TWENTY-TWO:	SEPARATION	76
MESSAGE TWENTY-THREE:	SENSITIVITY	79
MESSAGE TWENTY-FOUR:	THE UNIVERSE	82

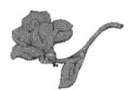

MESSAGE ONE

CREATION

You, me and everything – we are Creation.

How does one know this?

By FEELING through our physical bodies, which are our vehicles on this earth plane. These feelings become knowingness, recognition and a great sense of connectedness with all – everyone and everything.

The best way to allow these feelings to resonate in your physical body and to be aware of what is happening is to be truly in sync with nature. Mother Earth is our comfort and guide – she blesses us. We need to give thanks and be joyous and passionate in her abundance.

When you awaken and rise with the early morning sunrise and meditate or just fully connect with the sun's energy powering its life force onto planet earth – BREATHE IN and FEEL that energy resonating with your whole being.

As I awake I have this beautiful situation where I watch the sun coming through the tree tops of natural Australian bush, rising in the east, up, up in the sky with great intensity. The rays of energy of these two suns – the spiritual shadow sun – now fully vibrating also, energises and warms my body, gladdens my heart and so I feel the feelings of gratitude, peace, abundance and joy. I meditate with these feelings and know I want to feel as much intensity in my body as possible, abundantly and joyously.

My life here this time, like many others, has had more than its measure of pain, struggle and sorrow living our Piscean roles. I have always been in gratitude for my times of respite to balance my emotionally torn, weary vehicle with nature and often have peace there. Now I recognise that the more I resonate with these feelings the more I can embrace abundance and joy.

What is it about nature that YOU resonate with? The sunrise, the rainbows, the storms, a walk on the beach early morning or evening? How many of us love working in our gardens, are passionate about flowers, trees or herbs? Take time to smell the roses, as they say - take TIME OUT - this is truly the BEST healing and balancing medicine on the planet. How is it that so many have "lost" their contact with nature and the feelings we can "embrace" within ourselves? The "robotic" human vehicle has become driven on automatic pilot in the competitive third dimensional world, and fear is the steering wheel of our human frame via our nervous systems. Our electro-magnetic energy field, connected to All-That-Is allows us to fast track in this lane in life until we become an accident about to happen.

Our health and well-being is our prime concern and responsibility and many of us are out-of-control, on automatic pilot, before the inevitable happens to bring us back to balance with ourselves and life. This is always best accomplished by taking time-out in nature – she is our great Mother in this life and the more we respect her, the more we respect ourselves and the incredible spark of energy that we are in the big plan and scheme of evolution.

Yes, you, me and everything – we are Creation – here together today, to co-create Heaven on Earth!

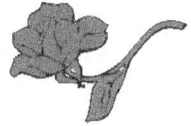

MESSAGE TWO

TRINITY

Father, Son and Holy Ghost.

The Sun rises from the East, from whence all new things come. Father, Mother and A Holy Child is Born. Maybe you were a first born? What excitement, what promise, what mission did you bring to earth to fulfil your soul?

The Holy Child was revered in ages past – the children of today are Angels on the planet – wise souls of vibratory energy who are radiated Beings, high enough to come through the energy grid of this evolving fifth dimensional planet. Those with Karmic or denser issues will not return to this earth to ensure that Heaven on Earth is fulfilled as creation's story.

Mother, Father and children of today. What amazing changes we are experiencing and we are all co-creating to fulfil earth's destiny. We heard the "call" and we are HERE!

Our Patriarchal Fathers always thought they were Supreme, the Masters, the Leaders and Controllers. Do they think that now? The Matriarchal Mothers of eons past were revered and respected and now the Balance of Male/Female energies are complete. We are all here to CO-OPERATE and

CO-CREATE together – not to compete and destroy anymore.

The name of the game is POWER WITH not POWER OVER – facilitating with Mother Earth and our genetic and spiritual families. Do you know why you came back here into your present family? As an incredible spark of energy, child of the Universe, mother or father, we each choose our beginnings and our destiny for our soul's mission and fulfilment. What incredible experiences are you attracting for your evolvement at this challenging time on Mother Earth? In three generations we awaken to the realisations of these changes.

When my father fulfilled his eighty-four years on earth this time around we acknowledged together what incredible changes he had experienced; from being the farmer who tilled the land with his team of draught horses, firstly as a boy alongside his father and then as a father himself, with his young daughter (me!) alongside him. His maturity years went from owning the first Model-T Ford car in the district to also being the first farmer to acquire the services of a helicopter to spray the land. He flew in an aeroplane to his genetic country of heritage – Scotland, the Celts, to fulfil part of his dream and adventure on earth.

He chose to be born into a traditional family with much Karma to be worked out, living in the country of the first light – New Zealand. His mother was Scottish and carried the Celtic genes of trust, loyalty and unconditional love, with the spiritual name Annie. His father came from the rugged shores of a fishing village in Scotland and became a pioneer farmer in New Zealand with a soft name, John, and a personality to portray him as hard, difficult and controlling. My father was the second born of nine children – they all experienced the first born being female and many Karmic patterns followed in their lives

In my awareness, as my father's second born child, I experienced these patterns flowing on into the next generation and am consciously aware of my own three children's significance with their present journey on Mother Earth. My second son now tills the land as a farmer, with tractors and bulldozers and his son sits in his spacesuit in the cabs! There has been recognition in New Zealand that the farmers are the backbone of the country and the Maoris are the fishermen – may all generations remember the blessings and abundance the land has given us and respect her. May the instinctive and patient nature of the Maori peoples never forget their ability as fishermen to protect and revere the waters of Aotearoa, where a marine park needs to be established in the aqua-blue Pleiades waters.

As we grow and mature we recognise our human backbone is the strength and security we have for our physical bodies to BALANCE ourselves with Mother Nature and life on this planet. Incorporated with this backbone is our CENTRAL NERVOUS system, our connector to and from the brain, our computer. In three generations we will see the imbalances mankind manifests and rectifies to balance ourselves and shift from the dross of the emotional Piscean era (Water) to mental (Aquarian - Air) clarity of living in the NOW in total harmony with All-That-Is.

Take care and nurture your MIND, BODY and SOUL of the third dimension as the physical temple, our body, makes these changes through cellular consciousness to fifth dimensional reality.

The "quickening" in energy on this planet, from years 1999 to 2012 is amazing and we are ALL new to the experience, however many lives we have had or however wise we are. We are to co-operate and support our fellow beings WITHOUT emotional attachment. MIND, BODY and SOUL is the TRINITY. In Universal Energy we are united in One Song.

FOOTNOTE:

If you do not think you need to cope with the changes, or your soul's mission is already fulfilled you are free to leave at any time! It is your choice - as choice is the biggest asset we have on this planet. I am too determined and stubborn to go yet, so I choose to be here to make sure we all get it together and
SING THE SONG!

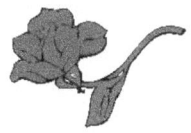

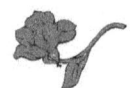

MESSAGE THREE

THE THIRD EYE

There is truly one mystery of life –the reflection of the mystery of self. What is self? Who is Self? WHO AM I?

The fear of the unknown is the biggest fear of all and when one does not enquire, wonder or marvel about self, one does not want to enquire and comprehend about life's possibilities, so therefore lack and limitations are life's order, instead of abundance and prosperity.

Life's explorations and mysteries are relevant in equal measure to the exploration and mystery of self. Who is self? What am I? I am a Spiritual Being having a physical experience. The all-knowing wisdom comes from the Third Eye – information from a multi-dimensional Being (self) here on earth, having an adventure in consciousness. I am the TRUTH! I am the WAY! I am GOD/GODDESS connected to ALL-THAT-IS – THE UNIVERSE – ONE SONG – WHOLENESS.

You are perfect. Whoever said you were not? Your mother, your father, your teachers, friends, society. Believe in yourself – this is your journey and you live your truth. We all know parts of the same truth but perception is the name of the game. What you perceive in the same situation or person is different from what I will or can perceive, therefore your truth is not necessarily my truth but we are all in the same story. We are all integral parts of the same matrix at present on earth co-creating Heaven-on-Earth consciously or un-consciously.

To be consciously aware is to be in LOVE, LOVE, LOVE with self and reflect this love in one's energy to all about us. We are the mirror – as within, so without.

To enjoy life's adventures is to enjoy one's uniqueness, idiosyncrasies, mysteries and mastery of self. We always attract what we most need to experience for our growth. Energy follows thought and when one's thoughts are fear based we will attract the experiences needed to overcome our fears with courage and self-love. Courage is the faith and belief in oneself – the flipside of FEAR. The more fearful the feelings you have felt and manifested from day one of your life until now, the more courage and belief in oneself one needs. You have it. We are each equipped with the necessary measures, as we do not attract more than we are capable of coping with. Where do these inner strengths come from in our times of great fears and miseries? From our higher selves (or inner selves) of all knowingness, our wisdom, our connection to All-That-Is.

The three aspects of living awareness that equip us, are our male and female energies balanced with our higher selves. Our Third Eye is the MASTER KEY.

When our two seeing eyes are closed our third eye opens, which is the reason why sleep, dreamtime, and meditation must be in balance with what we "see" on the earth plane. Close the eyes and FEEL the feelings. Your physical body is a transmitter of energies. Hands-On-Healing is an effective way to an understanding of self. To know one's self is the greatest mystery of life. To unlock the hidden aspects of your multi-dimensional self use your master key – the THIRD EYE. The challenge of life is to challenge one's self.

Close your eyes and feel the feelings of PEACE and DIVINE LOVE WITHIN. BREATHE DEEPLY and SLOWLY. THINK only PEACEFUL and POSITIVE THOUGHTS – you are a DIVINE BEING.

FOOTNOTE:
   A tool for the Third Eye development is a
     TIGERS EYE CRYSTAL.

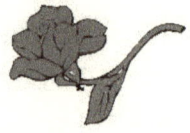

MESSAGE FOUR

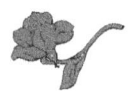

HERITAGE

You were born UNIQUE, SPECIAL and WONDERFUL.

It is your birthright to be abundant and prosperous. What has happened to your reality? Our genetic heritage is our foundations of this life. What family did you choose to come into and the unique, special and wonderful mother form that birthed you into the earth plane? When I first heard it said that I chose my mother I was incredulous. Oh No! I responded, I would have chosen any of my friends' mothers but not mine. At that time I was more aware of my mission on the earth, although my mother had been gone out of this life for nearly thirty years. I realised I was still carrying my mother's anger, sadness and discontent with life. Why had she been so resentful and judgemental when she died with a cancerous condition at forty four years of age? My little, older sister had died of leukaemia at three and a half years of age and my mother had never forgiven herself or God for her loss.

From two years of age I was to learn to be a good survivor and to this day I give thanks to my mother that due to my heritage I am as courageous as I am. There is as much about our parents that we most definitely do NOT want to do in this life as there is goodness that is our mirror to be like them. Our families are our foundations and for most give us the biggest challenges to experience ourselves on all levels - emotional, mental, physical and spiritual. The more we are challenged on these levels the more our experiences will empower us to react or respond to the bigger family of life. We are each unique, special and wonderful aspects of energy and an incredible part of the whole matrix of humankind on the planet.

What is your uniqueness and creativity that you are manifesting as a catalyst for change? This earth plane is an amazing school of life and there are no failures, only Karmic experiences - imprinted from our genetic foundations which we learn from to complete our soul's evolvement, mission and fulfilment. When you understand and know this you will be in gratitude for your parents and the reasons you chose to be part of those family foundations. Where resentments and bitter judgements remain, the human body will be distorted and life accordingly. Love energy is what makes the world go round and moves us into higher and brighter vibrations. When we release our energy blocks in our physical vehicle (temple) we are free to choose our path of least resistance and respond to life and it's challenges.

How is your vehicle – weary and worn, bitter and twisted or fully charged with super octane love power? Some of us have replaced many parts, maybe even the engine (the heart) during these days of clever technology. For a quick fix anything and everything seems possible. I have a new "team" to function in my mouth, to enable me to smile more happily, eat less and talk more slowly, as the "use-by" date was up with the old teeth.

Foundations are an important, inherited part of this life. The imprint in our cellular memories can be detrimental until we become aware that change is the only certainty. We can and must do our own self-love empowerment to enable our soul's mission to be fulfilled and ultimately know we have the power to choose what that is. Then we attract to us the situations, people and experiences that support rather than hinder our progress and mission.

Do what is your heart's desire. Live your passion and your creativity will enhance and enrich all about you. You are a shining light, a spark of energy come to be an amazing catalyst for change at an amazing time on planet earth.

If your foundations were limited you will either be inclined to stay limited too, or be the real catalyst (or rebel) for change that you are and UNLIMIT YOURSELF COMPLETELY. ABUNDANCE and PROSPERITY
IS YOUR BIRTHRIGHT!

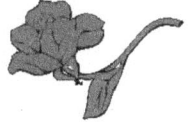

MESSAGE FIVE

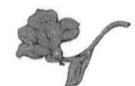

ATTITUDE

It has often been said that life is one per cent action and ninety nine per cent attitude - how we respond to every situation. It is also accepted that our bodies react or respond to everything and every substance - from water to alcohol, every food from organic fruit to red meat, every supplement and medication, and drugs - poisonous or otherwise. However, how can it be that some foods, medications, etc. can enhance some people's bodies and be detrimental to others? We are all different in our metabolic make-up and whatever we are thinking will determine our attitude, so in every given now moment our reaction or response can be different also. This is how our attitude determines an outcome and brings about our reality.

Awareness of self is the key to understanding this profound patterning, locked into our subconscious from birth and maybe lifetimes before. Energy follows thought and as we live on a loving, giving and nurturing earth planet, our lives ought to reflect that mirror. Energy is the life-force of the human body and everything about us. We are all energy beings. The problematic area, where anything and everything can go "wrong" and seem to be so difficult, is due solely to our FEARS - fears from childhood, from our parents, society and life's experiences. Anytime our body has reacted, we are running on the fear adrenalin. It's OK. We can survive. Many of us have had nervous systems geared to keep our bodies going, programmed by our fears since day one! Fear, like anger, can be a good energy as long as we are aware of our reactions and teach ourselves to change our thoughts, which is attitude and RESPOND to each situation instead.

The only certainty is change, so let us help ourselves by consciously making those changes ourselves and being in our power. We have incredible choice on this planet – choose to react OR respond and if at first you do not succeed you will always be given the opportunities to try again, as our experiences remind us what we have not mastered in ourselves. Like attracts like and we will attract the people, relationships and situations to enable us to make the changes that are necessary for our soul's growth.

Communication is a key factor to our success in life. How do you communicate? When insecure feelings take a hold of your tongue or your body, your body language still transmits to others what you are thinking. LISTEN to your thoughts. Take time out to contemplate and meditate and LISTEN to yourself. TUNE IN to your computer, the brain and/or mind and know that you are not just your physical body.

We are multi-dimensional energy Beings resonating to the Universal Mind of God. What is your special message coming through? At times, when the "static" is so heavy that you cannot hear or tune in, then tune out to yourself again and use a simple and powerful affirmation like "I AM LOVE", "I AM

BOUNTIFUL", "I AM IN ABUNDANCE", "I FORGIVE MYSELF FOR ALL THAT I HAVE ATTRACTED", "I RELEASE ALL I DO NOT WANT OR NEED ANYMORE", etc. Whatever is appropriate at the time, say it over and over until you not only believe it's possible – you know it. The feelings transmitted will confirm in you when they are positive and comfortable feelings and your listening skills are working.

Living our life on the fear adrenalin is being an accident about to happen with our health and/or experiences. However, we also are attracting those experiences to learn more about ourselves for our soul's growth and our mission here. So, with our thoughts we can change every difficult situation into a plus for ourselves. Out of every adversity comes the SEED of a greater benefit. Many a time I have said "When I know what the greater benefit is I will nurture my seed well" and many a time – on hindsight – I have discovered those greater benefits.

Serenity, patience and faith in oneself is our salvation. May I have the serenity to ACCEPT the things I cannot change, the COURAGE to change the things I can and the WISDOM to know the difference.

Courage has always been a key factor in my life. I know it well from de-programming my fears. However, serenity and accepting are bigger challenges for my development now and wisdom is most definitely the ultimate.

Maturity is experience – BE WISE!

MESSAGE SIX

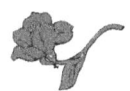

RESPONSIBILITY

Matriarchal influence has always had powerful strengths and capabilities to maintain responsible societies. Now, in these rapidly changing times, breaking down and through genetic coding, it is obvious that female power is being activated to fuller measures to bring about balance and responsible communities again. The subtle, helpful woman or partner behind the scenes is now OUT FRONT.

In my younger days I used to hear the phrase often said, "Behind every good man is a good woman." Then as a wife myself I acknowledged that alongside every good man was a good woman. In this next generation I know that in front of every good man is a good woman! Do the male species want to follow? That is their challenge, as they chose to be men in this lifetime. By following the direction – and/or examples – of the female goddess energy, men are able to nurture and listen to their own female goddess energies within for their own balance and direction.

The co-operation, harmony and peace needed on this planet can only come through each individual focussing on their worth or measure of male and female balance and peace within themselves. The goddess energy of enlightenment is allowing us to become unburdened of heavy patriarchal control and power-over tactics, to be lighter and brighter in all we think and do. Let us bring on the laughter and the angels to assist us! Until we accept the lessons that guarantee power WITH each other we cannot function in our societies happily and successfully.

Our creative uniqueness, abilities and strengths manifest through our sensitivities and emotions. Every man, woman and child is capable of being a genie, activating their own special brand of genius ability. How do you respond and use your abilities? The more we master our own unique abilities the more we are an asset to co-creating life on this planet.

Who are your mentors that show you their good qualities? They are often a grandmother or mother - within three generations. They are there as each family has their guiding lights on earth, who are usually big catalysts for change - either actively or subtly.

One of my favourite families on earth is the Royal Windsor family of England. It is so profound to see the matriarchal strengths of the women flow from the influence of the Celtic, strong Queen Mother, living here until one hundred and one years of age, through to her daughter, Queen Elizabeth II, considered to be the most powerful woman in England. The genetic flow through to Princess Anne, who has broken many traditional patterns, and Princess Diana, who has been the biggest catalyst for change with the Goddess energy, which opened the heart chakra energy grid of

England, with the outpouring of love and compassion after her dramatic life and tragic death.

These examples are all part of our lives as we reflect similar family patterns in the shift and re-balance of male/female, God/Goddess energies. The daughters (usually the eldest) take on the responsibilities that were their father's lot, especially when there is unfinished business to be attended to. The sons will have the goodness of their mother's and grand-mothers' energies flow to them, as love and compassion. Then creative abilities from within themselves are enhanced. In three generations we can comprehend the matrix of family life and the shift of abilities and power.

We are all the microcosm of the macrocosm and totally reflect the Big Picture, the Big Family of Humanity. We are each a unique part of the jigsaw puzzle, as at soul level we choose the families we were born into to learn and know how to respond to our abilities, to be more responsible in our lives and society, sharing our goodness.

RESPOND to your ABILITIES!
To CARE and SHARE is LOVE!

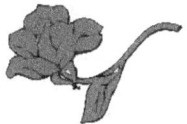

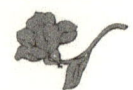

MESSAGE SEVEN

DIVINE WISDOM

What is the difference between wisdom and divine wisdom? Is there a different explanation for each? I believe and know there is. Wisdom comes from experience of doing-ness on one's journey. Divine wisdom comes from conscious connection to All-That-Is – the ability and power to speak and act from your higher self, intuition, Divine will. LET THY WILL BE MY WILL and MY WILL BE THY WILL. This recognition and acceptance comes from your inner knowingness of self on many levels, past lives included. Often the recognition starts when at ones lowest ebbs in life and searching "OUT THERE" for the knowledge and wisdom seems fruitless or more confusing. Then with feelings of doubt, sadness, insecurity and lack of love we will take TIME OUT with ourselves to GO WITHIN and love ourself, one's inner child, and nurture ourselves back to a new and stronger level of balance with All-That-Is.

When the beauty and power of ourselves is felt and acknowledged our connection as SPIRIT, GOD/ GODDESS energy resonates more fully and our Divine Will is stronger and more knowing. This is a time, when as a physical being we know we are spiritually guided and supported by the Universe. Many of us know we are receiving information via the Universal Mind, which is often called channelling – [being a channel, a messenger, a transmitter of energy for balance from heaven to earth.] Peace, love and praise needs to be activated for ourselves by ourselves to be able to proceed on our journeys in Grace - to JUST BE the "I AM" PRESENCE on earth.

Now, as I write I come from a "space" of maturity, having had amazing, exciting and devastating experiences during my present life here on earth and am truly capable of speaking and writing and sharing my feelings.

The secret is to master our fears and know that anything is possible when our WILL desires. Timing is the Universal trickster. How many times have you been sure that it is your luck to receive that which you desire and have used your abilities of prayer, affirmations, statements of purpose and more to no avail it seems! In the Big Story there is no TIME, as we know it now, which limits us accordingly. As we are each and every one an integral part of an immense jigsaw puzzle, we often have to "wait" until the "pieces" (people and situations) are in place, on our paths first. This is called PATIENCE and is perhaps the most profound and significant attribute of wisdom. Patience that all is in DIVINE RIGHT ORDER, patience to SURRENDER and TRUST, patience with our families and others, patience to LISTEN, patience to ACCEPT and be DETACHED from the outcome.

Those of us who have exhausted others by our demands and running on our nervous adrenalin will find patience difficult to master. The "panic buttons" that have been pressed in our earlier years due to the fear processes, have become our fight or flee survival aids. It is advisable to have trusted members of your family or friends who can remind you that you are "too much" in their energy space and you can "back-off" and mind your own business! Become detached and have more patience with self firstly and then others.

What is illness and time out in hospital for example – just an opportunity to learn patience with oneself and GO WITHIN to understand your own Soul's Path and Journey. I can reflect on those devastating times in my life as being of great value, as Out of every Adversity comes the seed of a Greater Benefit and when you discover that seed, NURTURE it for all it's purpose.

Ask and You Shall Receive. How many of us have not grasped that giving and receiving need to be in equal measures. We are here on this earth plane to work in togetherness. Coming together is a beginning, keeping together is progress and working together is success.

It all starts with the initial family and then the greater family of mankind. We are part of the Master Plan of evolvement of planet earth. We each chose to be here with our divine creative energy as the spark and missing link for many situations. We are each a catalyst for change, remembering always it is your own soul's growth that attracts all on your path. There are over six billion people on this planet and I know they will not all "cross-my-path" or meet me on this journey this time but those that do are all relevant to my soul's mission. I know I am an incredible catalyst for change - both within myself and WITH OTHERS. Let us love ourselves, have compassion for humanity and get on with it! I am running out of TIME to do my bit and I need your co-operation!

Stimulate your metabolism for more perspective and understanding, especially if you are over-sensitive and reactive, to stabilise and allow your shift from the emotional to the rational. Clear and still the mind to understand one's self and situations by releasing old mental patterns from the subconscious to allow for CONSCIOUS thinking. This is what our 'SHIFT" in the Big Story is all about - moving from the emotional feeling body of the Piscean Age to the mental, sensitive energy body of the Aquarian Age.

Spontaneity, ESP, and clear sight give us clarity.

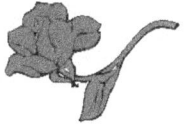

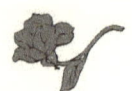

MESSAGE EIGHT

BALANCE

There comes a time in our lives when all that we thought we were, does not seem to really fit with all that seems to be! It is a paradox, our Pandora's Box of tricks because until we each individually and privately seek answers from within ourselves, we are searching outside of ourselves, often in vain. Why is this so? We have come into a life of separation and pain for the feelings of that experience. "Not good enough" or "better than" has been an ego or personality trait, which has brought about lack of self-love and self-esteem or workaholic individuals, always attempt-ting to prove they are good enough.

Competition has been the name of the game, instead of co-operation and appreciation of our own and therefore everyone's worth. We are really only competing with ourselves and proving that we are today better than we were yesterday, due to our attitudes and experiences.

Well I remember the day when, after nine years of breeding and training the best horses possible, I "made it" to the top with a champion horse. My vision and statement nine years earlier, when criticism and judgement was all about me, was "I'll have these horses at the top of the show world within ten years" and when I acknowledged that within myself nine years later, after many successful horses, my intuition/ higher self replied "Now that you have accomplished that and proved it to yourself, do you want to go on breeding and training horses to prove to others too?" My ego/personality accepted another of life's lessons of acceptance and my self-esteem was fortified in recognition of myself and my capabilities (which were cope-abilities against the odds!).

Being out of a good marriage, managing on my own with three children and thirty three horses, more often with the "odds against" me it seemed, I had challenged myself to my own vision and won. Only self-recognition was needed to fill my heart space with love. I had lived my passion of thirty odd years and my expertise and self-discipline had achieved my vision. Time had come to change my vision statement and move on as the soul yearns for more experiences!

Are you living your passion right now? What is your soul yearning to experience? The ego/personality is our helping friend that has the courage to act when fearful - love it, play with it and all its idiosyncrasies. Our soul is the messenger for our own truth and when we infuse the energies of personality to soul and soul to personality our BALANCE is our CHARACTER that keeps us all together – MIND, BODY and SOUL.

Balance with All-That-Is can be truly achieved when we are balanced in the moment, with all that we are. Often our imbalances distort our vision due to doubt, insecurities, depression and fears, however COURAGE is the Master Key and when capable of listening to self – the soul will speak to you for your passion to be lived. Some "moments" in time we are balanced, some "moments" we are not – that is life in duality, as we have always lived this life on an earth plane of polarities. GOOD/BAD, MALE/FEMALE, UP/DOWN, LIGHT/DARK, YIN/YANG. Due to the polarity we can know the success stories within and without us.

A lot of our balance in life comes from PURIFICATION - purification of our physical bodies and accordingly our thoughts. This is a process of RE-LEASE – releasing the old, stale, used stuff that does not serve us any more. After many experiences of cancer in my physical body (genetically coded for soul purpose) I am very aware of the re-leasing processes. My theory is that there is no such thing as "perfect health" as we are always in a process of change and the physical body is processing these changes in every moment. When we are aware and listening to our bodies we can "read" ourselves to understand what's happening better. Do not search for the perfect health from your doctor or health specialist or the many types of "fix you" people. They are just support in your process of change and you must know from within what support you require and know also that you always have CHOICE. There are incredible possibilities/opportunities for you from hands-on-healers to "New Age" technology. When in control of our own imbalances by taking responsibility for them, then have compassion with self or laugh at yourself to lighten your energy and then go about remaining in control of your own processes and power to choose what support you require.

Women have always been the natural nurturers, as the female hormones are equipped to cope, so women supporting women is a profound healing process. Most men love to be boys with toys, so the computers and technology of our times seem to be their forte! Do not ask them to come from their feelings or their hearts until they are ready to respond and learn from women! Why do you think that men can so easily have heart attacks – their heart chakras are obviously not functioning well.

In our "processes" of change and ill-health (ILL = I LACK LOVE) the feelings of nurturance, support and depth of understanding from those supporting us is far more valuable than technology that treats our bodies like machines with parts, instead of a spiritual being having a physical experience. Value yourself as such and treat yourself accordingly.

Mothers in this land, Australia, be aware as to what is happening with your children. They have chosen YOU to make these CHOICES for them – YOU have the power and freedom of choice for them and they are here as highly evolved spiritual beings to let you know medical propaganda must be avoided. They are the third generation (The Third Wave) to bring about the complete BALANCE of Heaven-On-Earth in this fifth dimensional shift of the planet. Be aware, LISTEN and take care of them, as they are the futuristic sparks of energy on this planet, radiating powerful energies.

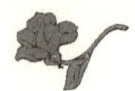

MESSAGE NINE

PATIENCE

It is patience with ourselves that will bring about our greatest healings. Patience is a poignant exercise, a lesson we will never stop learning, and as the more we excel in this attribute, the more humility we obtain.

I have had a feeling that I came into this life with an Aries attitude (from my previous past life) that portrayed an energetic busyness to get everything done as quickly as possible - that my message to the family and those around me was "Quick, Quick, this is how it is done or should be - let us get on with it so I can leave this planet again!" The problem was that no-one seemed to want to do it my way or be in such a hurry! I remember as a child often saying to my mother "I know there's a better place than this and when I have found it I am not coming back!"

Well, Out of Body Experiences and thoughts of ending my life have been options but through all that I am still here. What brought about these experiences of mine was total frustration - frustration with myself and with others due to the lack and limitations that seemed to be all about me. A difficult relationship with my strict mother and ten years of discipline from boarding schools taught me how to be a rebellious survivor. My survival issues taught me how to be courageous and stand in my own power as a woman with a soul's mission to fulfil, here on planet earth in these amazing times. It is recognised that there are more old souls on the planet now than there ever has been, starting with the one hundred and forty four thousand mentioned in the Bible, representing all races, tribes and creeds that have inhabited earth before. Those of us who came in and were born in the nineteen forties came into heavy dross energies from the nasty war that was meant to end all wars. These souls were part of the flower-power movement in the nineteen sixties, acting out their free will and freedom - who then became the leaders of the light in the nineteen eighties and the catalysts to work through generations of Karmic patterns in the nineteen nineties and finally fully Walk-Their-Talk and know the way in the New Millennium.

In my experience I have witnessed many wonderful women shine their lights and show me the way – they have been my mentors. I love the ditty that says "Patience is a Virtue - possess it if you can – seldom in a woman, never in a man!" Perhaps that explains a lot, as it has been mooted that most men (remember they chose to be men this time!) are five to ten years behind women in this shift of energy on the planet and can only "get-it-together" in understanding themselves by following or learning from women. Very scary for men I would say, as their number one fear is fear of women – usually starting with their mother. Mind you this scenario is also scary for women as their number one fear is fear of power, usually their own power.

So, how does patience work for us all? I believe it is the ultimate answer to be able to cope better and understand each other on all levels. When we are patient with ourselves and our soul's mission here we can be more patient with others, be able to discriminate, detach from and realise that we are all unique and wonderful, acting out a special part as a creative spark of the whole.

It is a certainty that all that we attract on our path – people and situations is for our experience, which usually requires measures of patience. I often say in my head, when feeling uncomfortable or frustrated, "that person is not on my wave length right now, therefore does not understand me" – then I detach and move on, minding my own business!

Patience with self enables us to have patience with others and life. Most of us are too demanding of ourselves, workaholics being the classic example, however when we look at the patterns that the subconscious mind is manifesting we will find the fears that motivate our behaviour – lack of self-love, self-esteem and not being good enough in some situation – family or workplace.

Patience with self becomes loving healing, and the humility that enables us to respond to others, not react. We are each at different stages of our learning and our missions – all in Divine-Right-Order.

As I write I have been in an incredible process with myself of SURRENDER and TRUST. For the past three years my busy-ness has become a being-ness that has enabled me to slow my pace, to be in a peaceful place and write. It has taken huge measures of patience with myself to achieve this moment in time.

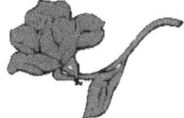

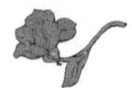

MESSAGE TEN

CHARACTER

I am the Caretaker of my Soul. My character is the sum total of my soul (inner self), personality (outer self) and all my multi-dimensional being ness. How many times have you heard the expression "Oh, she's a character", inciting the enthusiasm and joy shining through a person. These bright characters lift our spirits and make our days richer as they meet us on our paths. Are you a real fun character too or has your enthusiasm for life waned? When we can live life as an adventure, firstly in the physical like little children who are so open to exploration, then mentally and emotionally, taking control and responsibility for our thoughts and actions, the totality of our character lives through our creativity.

Our creative expressions and actions can seem like gifts from gods and we can fulfil our soul's mission. We are here in consciousness to express and expand – our physical vehicle, being the temple or house of our soul. Nurture your vehicle/temple and you can shine your light with grace. Think of a miner going into the mine shafts – he cannot see his way or do his work if his light is not shining bright. To see through our own darkness is to become night and day unified – what we think, what we dream, how we travel by night (astral) or day (vehicle) is an expression and expansion of our creative being ness.

In numerology terms my name, which represents our character, is a number nine, the humanitarian who wants to know and see it all. It was also the number of Jesus Christ, therefore a very challenging mission on the earth plane. The flip side (negative) of the number nine is that survivability comes through pain and suffering. Jesus Christ died at thirty-three years of age - thirty-three is the Master Number of Universal Service.

My thirty-third year of this life was my most memorable, when it seemed like I was living the life of my dreams with husband, family, extended family, horses and social fun. We are changing the coding, the genetic patterns for a life of adventure and creative expression. When security with my family was threatened and severely tested during the following three years I was able to use courage to manifest my creative expression and continue with my life of adventure. With hindsight, had I continued to live my life in a complacent manner with someone else wanting to control my character, I would not have experienced life's adventures the way I have and am so much wiser for being in my own power. We always have choices.

Do we have a destiny - a blueprint map that ensures we do what may not seem to be possible or feasible at times? I believe so, as we are each here to be and act as catalysts for change - all life is full of changes and choices. This too, often makes for insecure moments as one may experience confusion and doubts and be unable to make the changes or choice that the character is given. When that becomes the situation you are not in your power and fear is your guide and friend. Go within, love your uniqueness and master the courage required to have the faith in yourself that can do anything you desire. Often timing seems to be a problem, as the Universal time is the trickster and our spirit friends our helpers, do not know time as we are experiencing it.

Focus on your passion, your dream in your heart and listen to your higher self's advice that personally guides you. How much do you truly listen to your inner voice - intuition, instead of others' advice? How much faith and positivity do you have in yourself, to be in your own power? Take time out to learn more about your inner strengths and knowledge with the many metaphysical teachings that are available to all these days - numerology, astrology, past lives, etc. Value yourself, invest in yourself - MAN/WOMAN, KNOW THYSELF. YOU ARE A UNIQUE, SPECIAL AND WONDERFUL CHARACTER.

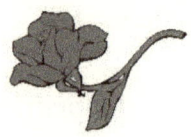

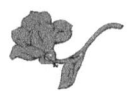

MESSAGE ELEVEN

RELAXATION

It is my natural state to be relaxed and at peace with myself at all times. To focus on the end result of my soul's mission on earth and know that all is in Divine Right Order. Oh, that I could live this state of well-being all the time!

We have all gone about as far as we can go with work, work and more work for the sake of the mighty dollar, without destroying the planet and ourselves. Enough is enough to recognise how out of balance we have been and our physical health will suffer due to the mental and emotional stresses. The key to good balance is equal measures of relaxation and time out from our work or career. Are you achieving this for the benefit of your health and well being?

Why is it so difficult for most people to relax? Their nervous systems are taxed to the max and their high-octane fuels is the fear adrenalin of fight or flee. Fear or love fuel the energies that drive our vehicles. Our life-force energy is pure love and becomes distorted or blocked when the fear energy takes over. To recognise and understand our fears and then to transmute them is the master key to relaxation and well-being.

How is it that most of us take days to "unwind" our robotic selves when on holiday and it is only just achieved when it is time to pack our bags again and go home and return to the robotic workplace. To be relaxed, allows our unique creativity to be actioned in a balanced and healthy way – we are each in the workplace to enhance it, not to be controlled by it. This is why so many people start their own creative businesses and may they continue to be successful for the sake of our country, the planet and ourselves.

It has been stated from many sources that Australasia leads the way for this new paradigm of the millennium as an example to the rest of the world. It is to be hoped that the energy generated in the year two thousand with the Olympic Games will be repeated often. Australia depends on small businesses for the well-being of it's people and the land. To avoid the multi-national power games, particularly from American influences (the Illuminati), people need to honour themselves living in this great landmass – OZ!

Be in your own power and know as a voting member you need to be open, aware and caring for the future of this wonderful country. Local communities are the essence of our soul's work, which is the reason why so many people have moved or retired to the smaller towns, where community caring and sharing is the essence of life. Relaxation can more easily be attained in these environments, enhanced by nature's wonderland of bush, landscapes, water, lakes, sea, wildlife and animals. Go walking in nature. To own a cat and/or dog is to enhance your ability to relax and play.

Relaxation seems almost impossible when pain becomes suffering. When discomfort is the norm in one's body and anxiety is the norm for one's mind, efforts to become relaxed can seem fruitless. This is when, with awareness one can self-discipline oneself and with a focus on the breath, breathe through the pain. When we have focussed on the breath and master it consciously we will eliminate all pain and suffering as pain in the physical body is only a reminder of an imbalance creating stress [dis-ease].

When the breath is used consciously by taking time-out and resting, the physical body re-balances itself more quickly. Often a healing crisis, when the body is making a dynamic effort to heal, is more painful than an accident crisis. Have you experienced that? Many people first take painkillers, drugs or alcohol to numb the pain but the pain is a message from the body that a process is happening that needs our attention and full focus on understanding ourselves metaphysically. The aches and pains of our physical bodies are messengers waiting to be decoded.

Relaxation is the essence and balance of all our healing processes. Breath is our prana, our life force energy. Those of us who use Reiki have a powerful adjunct to help us through our times of pain and imbalances. Reiki is the energy of life, in the spirit of love. The more we love ourselves and our transgressors, the easier and quicker the healing – just forgive ourselves for what we have attracted for our experience and wisdom will be the outcome.

Music is a valuable asset in times of stress and healing - always have your favourite music handy on tape or CD, to play at such times, especially when you are unable to sleep. Soothing, relaxing music will calm the nervous system and the mind - your computer needs to be turned off for a while.

Life is a challenge on the earth plane – a school of life. When one accepts that the thorns are as much a part of life as the roses, we can manage our health processes better and master our well being. Good practitioners can support us to help and understand our processes better. To relax is to enjoy life and know that all is in Divine Right Order. Mind, Body and Soul are in harmony, working together as our orchestra and we are our own conductor.

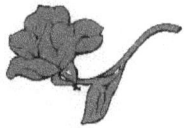

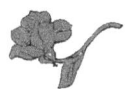

MESSAGE TWELVE

CREATIVITY

Creativity is the manifestation of your uniqueness, abundance and prosperity. Often, without recognising your uniqueness it will manifest from your passion – the enthusiasm that drives your 'Being' into action.

Our will is the most powerful motivator of all, as it is our deepest desires from within our soul. It comes from the divine – let my will be thy will. Connected to All-That-Is, our soul manifests through the will, our creative gifts and expertise (from past lives) to act. Creative manifestation is both constructive and destructive, as action can be constructive or destructive because we live in a world of polarity. Often, when Karmic influences are strong, we need to be part of the destruction (breaking down) before there can be new construction for better ways of being and living.

To love our idiosyncrasies, we need to love the dark side of ourselves – the so-called bad, the devil, the trickster who as an aspect of us is part of our persona, to act as a catalyst for change on this planet. I admire those who have often been judged for their so-called "bad actions" when acting as part of destructive energies, breaking down old ways in society, for new ways to come through. On hindsight, many such courageous people have been recognised for their goodness.

Often one needs to be very brave to live one's passion, one's mission on this earth. Often, we are unable to manifest our creativity without the aid, co-operation of others, so frustrations can turn to anger or hopeless-ness, when timing does not synchronise. As the Universal timing is now quickening, there is recognition of being more aware of our consciousness levels and finding that synchronicity is working much better and quicker for us. This is mainly due to attracting others on the same wavelengths onto our paths.

Often, when I feel uncomfortable in the presence of another, I will say in my mind "this person is not on my wavelength right now and does not understand me" – then detach from that situation. There may come another time when our paths cross again and I will know we still have unfinished "business" together, as we are all here connected to learn from each other and work together in co-operation and compassion, to bring about harmony, balance and unconditional love.

We are created in the Creator's likeness and Jesus' words were "greater things than I, will you do" so after two thousand years plus we ought to be able to do that! What is "THAT" you may wonder? It starts with living your passion, having the courage to believe in your capacity, to act out your soul's mission, then be able to comprehend that we are all in the Big Picture together – the good and the bad, through difficult and easy times.

To make our lives easier we need to change our attitudes – towards ourselves, others and situations. By making light of our own work, laughing at our past adventures and ourselves. We can love our idio-syncrasies!

It is a recognised fact that the funniest comedians that offer their creative gifts to lift up others' spirits have usually come through the saddest and deepest traumas for their soul's growth and are acting out the opposite polarity. Their lightness and fun is beneficial to and for others.

Creativity is mind, body and soul working together for the greater good of mankind – either destructively (to break down) or constructively (to break through) into new foundations. Life is always changing and we are all manifesting these changes with our creativity. Creative gifts are not just sewing, knitting and cooking, etc. but are the totality of our uniqueness that has the ability to move over the rocks and climb the mountains.
What you perceive in yourself and what you believe you can achieve, you will – your Will will act through your soul's passion. Live your passion and release your potential for the benefit of mankind on planet earth.

There are wonderful examples and mentors on this planet, including the Queen Mother who has recently left the planet after one hundred and one years of living her passion and giving service with strength, dignity and laughter. The Queen Mother had a Master Life Path Number, to live a life of greatness to the benefit of mankind. When born with Master Numbers, greater things than I, will you do.

Have yourself a mentor or a "pin-up" as a mirror to encourage you to use your own inner strengths and abilities to leave your mark also. We are all equal but at different stages of our own journeys.

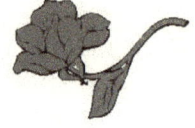

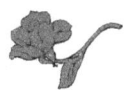

MESSAGE THIRTEEN

CO-OPERATION

Co-operation comes from an understanding of com-passion. When one is acting compassionately with oneself, an attitude of co-operation is attained with the ultimate results being our innate power in harmony WITH other BEINGS. The opposite polarity of power OVER other beings comes from control which is fear based. When our own being is running on the fear adrenalin we cannot be motivated to act in true co-operative spirit, but instead we will attempt to control others and situations.

This unfortunate process has nearly always planted its roots firmly in family upbringing - there always seems to be someone wanting to control someone else, or everyone in families. Firstly, the patriarchal father or the matriarchal mother, then their children grasp the idea with their own fear adrenalin and decide - usually unconsciously - to control others also. The bottom line of this behaviour is the controlling person not FEELING good enough about themselves and afraid of having their perceived inadequacies found out. The positive aspect is when praise is given in a loving manner from fathers and mothers, children will FEEL good about themselves and the seeds of self-love will continue to flourish with growth.

When the self-love process has not been established in childhood, particularly during the first seven years and the fear process has rooted itself into the child's psyche from the fear of someone else having control and power over them, this will flow on into adulthood.

Fortunately for the female of the species, our hormones are very expressive in a nurturing way and our efforts to become more co-operative in all situations with all people will extend with the measure of self-love and compassion we have for ourselves.

How can one possibly fully co-operate with others – give and take – respect and value in equal measures, when one does not value and respect their own uniqueness and creative talents? Wanting to be in control of others and situations all the time limits others and limits us. When one is able to surrender and trust in the Universal Divine Flow of Energy, which we are all part of, the understanding of co-operation from compassion becomes easier to comprehend.

Adjusting from controlling others due to fear related motivation to co-operation WITH others from compassion is the grass roots of the changes that are being made in all families and peoples now, to work together in a harmonious world. We know that the more powerful people become the more power they assert. When it is motivated by fear and control, misery is usually the outcome. When motivated by love and compassion – humanitarian aspects and acts will be the results. This simple truth is a profound key of change for our times not only for survival of ourselves but also the planet earth. S.O.S. = Save Our Selves, Save Our Souls!

As we act with co-operation with an attitude that benefits others, so we are able to act in co-operation with Mother Earth to bring about better balance of our earthly domain.

Life without co-operation becomes our Hell-On-Earth. Hell-On-Earth derives from jealousies - jealousy derives from lack of love. When a jealous person acts competitively, fear-based control is the name of the game. When this manifests in a species we have wars. Women do not create wars - women must lead the way with their co-operative natures and capabilities to bring about more peace.

Peaceful results come from a peaceful attitude that has its roots in self-love in the heart. When peace is within us we will be able to bring about peaceful results, with co-operation and compassion.

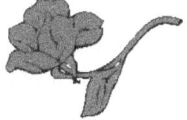

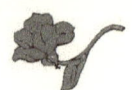

MESSAGE FOURTEEN

PAIN

Without pain we would not know struggle and without struggle we would not know how to make our lives easier and more full of love.

From an unexpected headache to the process of dying to a part of ourselves – pain is part of our experiences on the earth plane. Pain is the opposite polarity to ease, therefore disease is what we manifest. However, pain is also a blessing in disguise and the sooner we accept our pain and acknowledge its message the easier our relief will be.

In my experience RE-LEASE is the name of the game, as we always have something to re-lease when pain is part of our lives. There are very few illnesses without pain in the physical body. The feelings of pain are the messages to us that something needs to be released – our being has an energy block that needs to dissipate. Reiki, massage and Touch-For-Health are wonderfully beneficial to understand our bodies and to comprehend the messages, so that we can consciously release the pain. There are many ways to release the pain – firstly with our comprehension of what attitude is causing our mental and/or emotional blocks and consciously using our breath. To breathe fully into the heart chakra, then slowly breathing out, down the whole body and changing the breathing pattern into a slow rhythm, which changes the auric (blueprint) energy of the body for easier release and healing.

The "poor me" feelings are a message to ourselves that a part of us is out of balance and needs our attention. A state of balance with the mind, body and soul working in harmony is the ultimate quest, as life is all about changes to process ourselves into a higher state of consciousness.

There ought to be no such word as "sick" as it seems to relate to the fact that we need to be fixed by someone else. I call it the dark night of the soul, when we need to understand ourselves better. There is no sense in looking for a fix from those who cut, burn or poison and have no understandings of holistic health or higher states of consciousness. In simple terms, this means, "Know Myself and Heal Thyself". Take time out, the body and mind just need rest, relaxation and rejuvenation. There are many less invasive methods of healing the body holistically and becoming more in tune with the whole self. Vibrational Healing is Energy Medicine, which is the medicine of the NOW and the future.

Impatience with ourselves is detrimental to our process. Allowing ourselves to be open to receive support from others, involves our lessons of humility and compassion with ourselves, to evolve more towards unconditional love.

My own pain and struggle in this life has brought me into a greater understanding of others so that my work in service as a healer, teacher and practitioner has more profound results. One can empathise with another to the extent of one's own experiences. True empathy does not come from academia, which is left-brain – it comes from intuitive knowledge, which is right brain. Our right brain is fuelled by our third eye and sees the whole picture – holistic. The left-brain then analyses that for practical results. The hypothalamus gland is the master key between the left-brain and right brain, which is hormonal. All our emotions are hormonally driven, which can make our lives confusing, not only for ourselves but even more so for those around us!

To direct the mind, the will – to understand and control the emotions is to achieve harmonious balance for the body. Only FEAR hinders the body from balance and its own innate ability to self-heal. Nurturance is love, faith in oneself, which is the opposite polarity to fear. Our soul's mission is speaking to us via our faith, love and charity to be who we truly are and render service on this planet.

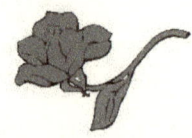

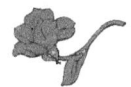

MESSAGE FIFTEEN

FUN

A young friend of mine recently stated that life is really just a play. Well, it's no wonder many of us seem to have been in dramas most of our lives! Let's just have fun instead.

To really be relaxed and enjoy life is to have no fear, a good sense of humour and be able to laugh at one's self. If life is just a play, then our persona (our outer self) is the masks we put on to play the roles, where we gain our confidence and courage. Our soul is our inner self and as we gain more confidence and courage we actually begin to live our lightness and brightness as a spiritual being, to manifest our soul's missions.

Laugh at our "worry-warts", laugh with others and Joy will become more infectious in our lives. How I love good party friends, who can always relate a funny joke or two and have me laughing until tears flow from my eyes. We need to be able to flow tears of joy, just as much as we can flow tears of sadness – that gives us our empathy, our love for self and others, our compassion.

Let us all make efforts to laugh more. To be joyous is to be bountiful, to FEEL prosperous and wealthy. Watch children and see how easily they play - we all need to play. What is your passion? Play with your passion.

One of my best playmates was my father. He could easily mimic others and would do so at a party to create fun and laughter amongst us all. I will go to a good movie if it is going to give me a good laugh, in preference to one that is full of emotional drama and sadness. If life is a movie I have had enough dramas without watching them on the big screen or television.

Whose drama are you involved in? Make sure it is of your own making, otherwise you may find yourself in someone else's drama and that can be very uncomfortable which results in you giving your power away - your true self will not be in alignment. When I experience that feeling I say in my head "mind your own business Rose-marie" and I move away!

There is so much in life to enjoy, especially watching young animals with their antics of play. Kittens and puppies bring a refreshing sense of joy. Never lose the ability to have fun and share laughter with many. Service can become a chore - lighten up with your laughter.

Life is a play - let's play with it.

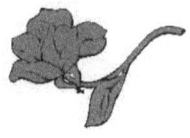

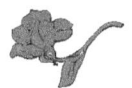

MESSAGE SIXTEEN

BEAUTY

Beauty is in the Eye of the Beholder.

Whether it be the beauty of a flower, the landscape, a painting or a china plate – all recognition of beauty is a reflection of self. Therefore, when one recognises beauty in another human being it is also a reflection of ourself – a mirror. Our mirrors in life are becoming more and more profound as we grasp the concept of our awareness of others, life and all things.

We attract to ourselves what we most need to learn from, for our soul's experience and often these situations can make us feel comfortable or very uncomfortable. This is the key of understanding energy. When these FEELINGS of discomfort concern us we are most likely to react. Connecting to the feelings from our body, mind and spirit, we can acknowledge HOW we are feeling and what we are thinking in the moment, as one's thoughts are the powerhouse. When our energy field becomes disturbed our bodies will feel uncomfortable. Our thoughts (which usually become words) distort our energy fields – as energy follows thought, therefore be aware of how comfortable or uncomfortable you FEEL in every moment, place and situation. When one feels uncomfortable just change your thoughts - your attitude and the circumstances will change also. The recognition of this ability and then the amazing results that manifest can enable one to be comfortable in situations we previously could not have coped with. As one changes one's thoughts, so the situations seem to change also. It is worth the effort.

I have always been greatly challenged in this life by recognising and coming to terms with my attitudes and thoughts. My first mirror in my life was my Mother who perhaps had the most critical and judgemental attitude of any person I have ever known – probably due to her own lack of self-forgiveness, self-love and self-esteem. My childhood and teenage years were difficult and the only way I seemed to keep my balance was to see the good in every person and situation. I had a happy-go-lucky attitude with my friends and all of life that consequently gave me the ability to laugh and play, therefore usually avoiding being uncomfortable.

Having had ten years at boarding schools, from six years of age, I was away from home and my mother for two thirds of those years and I learned to develop a good fun personality because when I was at home during holidays my life was always uncomfortable due to the fear adrenalin that came from our family home.
In later years I recognised how I had locked away my feelings of frustration, anger, anguish and sadness that ultimately helped create the cancerous conditions in my body. To unpollute my mind, body and soul from this mess I

learnt to love the beauty in nature more and therefore loving the beauty in myself more.

Hate is such a forceful opposite polarity to LOVE, and so the mirrors will teach us to have compassion and love for ourselves more. Competitiveness usually brings about jealousies that I believe bring about the evils of the world with the POWER OVER others situations.

Fear is such a powerful opposite polarity to FAITH as the mirrors will teach us to have faith in ourselves more, know and love ourselves as a unique, special and wonderful spiritual being in human form.

Beauty is in the eye of the beholder – you are the beholder.

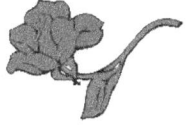

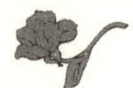

MESSAGE SEVENTEEN

ADVENTURE

Among my flowers I have come to see life's miracles and it's mysteries.

Life has it's miracles as well as it's mysteries – the mystery of life is an adventure. To truly live in the NOW present moment, is to trust the Universal flow of energy. We are Divine Spiritual Beings having a physical adventure as part of our journey here on the earth plane. All is in Divine Right Order.

We are, each and every one of us, an intrinsic part of the matrix of evolution, a part of the jigsaw puzzle of a never-ending mystery. Without worry or any anger we can enjoy our creative expertise.

What are your strengths and assets that you have brought here from other lives and other realms? Do you recognise the catalyst for change that you are, here on Mother Earth? What are your thoughts that are your friends or your enemies? What good ideas, inspiration has come through your third eye this morning to start a new day of adventure? In this life of polarity I have always had enlightening ideas of how I can turn the minuses into plusses and the miseries into positive outcomes for myself and for the benefit of others. We make the changes in ourselves when we know everything can be changed. Life is change, it is movement, it is vibration. The only certainty is change. How flexible are you?

I used to be so frustrated by people who changed their minds when I thought decisions were made to keep semblance of order – control seemed necessary. Now, I acknowledge that the unexpected changes in my life have brought me the greatest challenges and the biggest adventures. To be flexible is to be open to possibilities – to affirm that anything is possible, instead of limiting ourselves.

As all control has the adrenalin of fear motivating it and as we are spiritual beings having an adventure on the earth plane, we have an innate desire to have freedom WITHOUT control.

By living our passions from our hearts, our creativity is free to express and expand in recognition of our soul's purpose. What is your soul's purpose expressing and expanding into now? The Universal timing is the trickster, as you may achieve your desires in one day, one year or one century! Your Blueprint or Map of Yourself is your governing factor and the messages to show the way come through your INTUITION. Have you unfurled your map lately, to get an inspiration of what may be around the next corner? Who knows what tomorrow may bring with it – opportunities or challenges or both? Be enthusiastic about each new day – it is another beginning.

How I love the saying "every cloud has a silver lining" (when my chips are down). Live each day with a sense of adventure, as if it could be your last.

I remember during my years of riding on the hunting fields, seeing a horse or his old master die of a heart attack. What an adventure they were having, living their passion and dying in the moment. It was always said by the most dedicated horsemen – they died doing what they loved the best.

We die to a part of ourselves every day. Our healings for transformation are most profound during the night when the physical body rests and the astral body resonates with All-That-Is. We awaken to rejuvenated cells and our memory consciousness is sparked with new fuel, new energy. Life is an adventure every new day! Do not wonder if you are making an impression on the world – marvel at the wonder of yourself, as everything you think, say and do makes an impression on the world. You vibrate energy that is connected to all and everything. We all make a difference and therefore are part of the changes of the earth plane – co-creating the adventure.

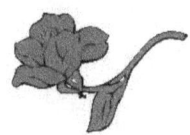

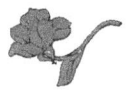

MESSAGE EIGHTEEN

FRIENDS AND FAMILY

A Friend.
Strengthens the heart, repairs the hurts.
Encourages the discovery, enlightens the mind.
Dissolves the pain, banishes the loneliness.
Understands the anxiety's, increases the joy.
Deepens the Spirit, frees the Soul.

My best and beautiful friend Raewyn died of cancer – she and I had had the most rewarding and happy relationship for many years. As mothers bringing up our children on our own, we supported and understood each other through all the promising good times and the challenging, difficult moments from the time our marriages fell apart. We were not at school together, when so many good friendships are formed but ironically met each other through our husbands, after we were married – they were best friends also.

After twelve years of married life with three wonderful children I found I was unable to remain married when my husband preferred to sleep and party with another woman. Such is often normal circum-stances for patriarchal relationships; however I was devastated as I had not anticipated such a situation.

As life is all about changes and challenges, this catharsis in my life was the second most significant loss after my mother's death with cancer just three years prior to my marriage. With no mother or husband for support (love and comfort), my father who had always been my closest ally, once again became my best and loyal friend – an incredibly strong friendship that we had until he left the earth plane at eight-four years of age.

My dear friend Raewyn's marriage ended after fourteen years, when she found her family situation too difficult to endure and with her four beautiful children, she also left the farming life to work and bring up her family in the same town as myself. With our seven young children we formed a friendship and bond of support that maintained our sanity and sense of humour for the forthcoming years – until she also died with cancer. We were so alike in so many ways that people often thought we were sisters. We formed a relationship of trust and support that became love and laughter at its best.

During my married years I had three sisters-in-law, all living in close proximity. As neighbours they were supportive and friends of great value. Between us all we were mothers of fifteen wonderful children, so our friendships were formed from understanding each others experiences as young mothers, women and supportive friends. These valued friendships that sustain us through changes and challenges in our lives are like our daily bread of life!

Always on our paths are these wonderful helpmates – some connect with us a little while and others keep coming back on our paths, which always gives me the feeling that we have more to understand from each other – usually the lessons of forgiveness. Unconditional love can be a big measure to really live as TRUST is such a big part of the equation.

When we live the experiences of friendship and support with our friends and neighbours, our levels of understanding can become so profound that uncon-ditional love becomes the ultimate desire. However, there is a master key to a part of ourselves that must be unlocked – the ability to receive in equal measure. Life is giving and taking. Life gives us breath to live and takes away our loved ones.

Women in particular, need to grasp the opportunities given to them to receive and open their hearts; otherwise the opposite polarity of resentment will keep the heart chakra guarded.

As women are natural nurturers, due to their hormonal functions, they often give plenty of nurturing and support to children, family and friends. Consequently, they become very depleted in themselves. To receive and give love unconditionally is to have one's own heart chakra full of self-love. We can only give out in equal measure to that which we have within ourselves.

My three best friends – my father, Raewyn, and my daughter – have taught me how to give and receive in equal measure, as we do not "owe" each other anything. The scales to balance our unconditional love with each other have been even and steady. I know my heart is open to receive now, from sources that surprise me, and from where I least expect it to come from.

The Universal Energy of Love is free flowing and unconditional.

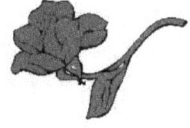

MESSAGE NINETEEN

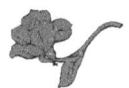

PRIDE

It is said that Pride comes before a Fall – pride is ego and ego is our personality. It is part of our Tool Kit in the playground of life.

Transcendence is the personality infused with soul and soul transcending personality – which simply means, as we become more aware of the roles the personality plays as our confidence booster, we find more courage to live our soul's message. The soul's mission is the primary purpose for which we each came to the earth plane, on this stage of our journey. The soul knows our creative expertise, our strengths and weaknesses. When our pride, [personality], has a setback in this life it is to remind us that our experience of humility, coming from our awareness of self, will have us resonating to our soul's message.

When people have a matter-of-fact attitude (casual) about an experience or situation, they are simply stating the "facts-about-the-matter" without emotional attachment because their own emotions have already played out the drama in a previous experience, which has given them the knowingness of their truth. For instance, when I can say as a matter-of-fact that cancer is easy to cure when you want to be cured, it is because I have lived through the experience and know the results are beneficial for my soul's mission. Like many others, I am a catalyst in the cancer story on the earth plane and like many others I have changed the genetic coding for the better, by bringing about more balance and harmony and by recognising how fatalistic the fear process can be in the cancer scenario.

Our energy of life is surely our breath, our life force and when lived in the spirit of love, all life has beneficial purpose. However, when the emotions coming from fear intervene, life becomes distorted and dis-ease can manifest. Faith being the opposite polarity, is our belief and faith in ourselves - self-love which keeps us in resonance with our soul's mission - our inner strengths, our capabilities, our passion, purpose and peace.

To follow through with our own spirit's messages requires confidence and courage and until we are all on the same wavelength (which is not likely to happen!) these attributes of doing-ness come from the pride personality.

Allow yourself to go as far as you can with confidence and courage, as life will give us each our lessons of humility in equal measures - pride comes before a fall. The fall is going within and understanding self from our inner depths. You may call these feelings sadness, depression, anguish - they are all part of the process of being a human BEING on this planet. The good news is that we are all waking up to this process which is accelerating in the higher energy field and so we do have others for support on our wavelength of intuitive understandings. Extra Sensory Perception, often called ESP, is our ability to connect with others on wavelengths that surpass the need for computers. Meantime, computers are the "bridge" to mankind's brain to recognise and adapt to this intuitive way of knowingness.

Wake up brains - we only use ten per cent of them - or is it one per cent? Do not be "hood-winked" by academia, as our creative genius abilities come from the right brain which sees the whole picture and is fuelled by our third eye, the intuition, our spiritual faculty. THIS is the information that keeps our soul's mission on track!

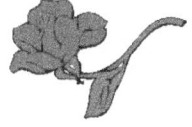

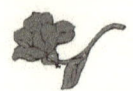

MESSAGE TWENTY

DIMENSIONAL SHIFT

THIRD.........FOURTH...........FIFTH - It is stated that we have been living a third dimensional existence on a third dimensional planet and now this planet is the last in the cosmos to move through into the fifth dimension. That, in fact, she is now in the Photon Belt of Radiation, which is giving humanity some big awareness issues and experiences.

To enjoy this transition of change is to master one's own balance without the fear process predominating. To go to extremes with feelings of sadness and joy has often been our experience. For example, the death of a loved one viewed as loss and sadness that we ought to celebrate in joy that the loved one is returning to source. We welcome a new birth with joy, when perhaps we could have compassion for this little soul who will be challenged with living in a body on the earth plane.

Limitations and lack disappear in the fifth dimensional energy, as all is abundance, joy and prosperity. Co-ordinating ourselves on all levels - mind, body and souls - is the process we are all partaking in NOW. This co-ordination becomes a re-evaluation and thus a realignment of the human form. A BEING and becoming that is true to our essence, our nature spirit, our source. The source is tangible and intangible, as it is within and without us – energy of All-That-Is.

We have become so used to some force having power over us and somebody else being responsible for us that the realisation that this shift into higher consciousness is entirely of our own making is our "wake up" call. No thing or person, teacher or guru is going to do it for us but we can be guided by the mirror of others who "Walk-The-Talk" and therefore lead by their example.

Using our intuitive expertise and opening our hearts to be vulnerable to all the possibilities on our path gives us an awareness so that we attract what we most need to learn from. Often this could be the opposite of what we have affirmed, because those experiences help us to have a firmer faith in ourselves and the courage to stay grounded in our own power.

I remember one of my earlier experiences with my horse stud when I was asked why I had called a young horse Challenge and I replied "because I am challenged by the opportunities that this young horse will give me while training him to learn more about the breed". He became a champion jumper, winning hunting awards for five years in a row. Consequently, I often say I have learned more from horses this life than I have from my fellow human beings! Their senses have five times greater perception than humans and their third eye capabilities are incredible when one understands them. They do not talk like humans, so one has to read their mind so to speak, to talk to them, and FEEL their feelings when riding them. It is no wonder that so many sensitive and emotional young people enjoy their ponies and horses – a unique partnership of trust evolves between them.

We all have experiences and "tools for our trades" that give us the perception to shift our awareness and therefore our energy fields into a higher vibratory dimension. I thank my lucky stars that one of mine is having had horses as friends all my life. Perhaps you have cats or dogs, donkeys or goats to empathise with too – I hope so!

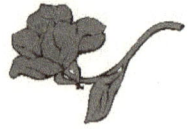

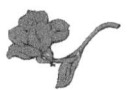

MESSAGE TWENTY-ONE

GRATITUDE

Gratitude is like love – we can never have too much of it.

I always thought I had appreciated the good in my life every day of my life but recently I discovered that as I had developed a much deeper awareness of feelings of gratitude for myself, I have come to appreciate the goodness in all things, large and small, even more.

> All things bright and beautiful
> All creatures great and small
> All things wise and wonderful
> The Lord God made them all

As we are matter in human form, formed from energy, our being-ness becomes our doing-ness. We are all Energy Beings, doing our creative work on the Earth planet. As such, we need to be in gratitude for ourselves for the creative energy that we are – becoming more capable, bright and beautiful, great and small, wise and wonderful, as co-creators to work and play on Mother Earth.

How come we have grown so serious, our personalities taking on a righteous attitude that we are not good enough? Often in the beginnings of our lives, when as children, the "Not-

Good-Enough" syndrome has often become the norm to keep us detached from our uniqueness and therefore degrading ourselves, compounded with a lack of self-love and self-nurturing, so that our journey here seems to be difficult rather than flowing with ease. Having all come through the Piscean Age may explain these experiences as the Piscean Cross representing Jesus' sufferings has emphasised the good/bad polarity greatly, especially in religious wars. The Aquarian Age is represented by the equal sided Aquarian Cross, which is similar to the original Celtic cross. The Hopi Indians predicted that when the white man came to them with the Aquarian cross they could then join in union, and peace with all peoples would become possible. This has happened. As we are all here to co-create in the Aquarian Age, the Thinking Communication Age, represented by the Water-Bearer, we are releasing the last layers of suffering in the memory consciousness of the body to realign with our higher consciousness and so go forward in gratitude. To give thanks to others is a happy feeling – to FEEL gratitude for self for just being the I AM is an even greater measure of love. We recognise we have each chosen to be here as a spiritual being in human form at this amazing time of changes and challenges from one dimensional age to another.

We are all now co-creating, firstly with our thoughts and as energy follows thought we manifest accordingly. The more like minds there are on the same wavelength with similar thoughts bring about manifestation more quickly, which is why group meditation is so subtly powerful. Peace can manifest with peaceful thoughts from a peaceful Being.

Having peace within oneself is usually a difficulty that is why to FEEL gratitude with self is essential. In a competitive environment to give and receive from others unconditionally is usually difficult due to uncomfortable feelings. With a co-operative attitude, without emotional manipulation, firstly amongst ourselves and then in society, we can all benefit from giving and receiving unconditionally with joy and ease, then the measures of gratitude for self will be enhanced.

Recognising goodness and beauty in nature and goodness and beauty in others is the mirror reflection of the goodness and beauty in self. The saying "It takes one to know one" is a truth.

By resonating in one's own truth, one remains in one's own power which enables us to give and receive in equal measure with joy and ease rather than guilt and discomfort. Always feel the feelings of the body in these situations and when uncomfortable, change your attitude with your thoughts and resonate with love in your heart. Does it give YOU a good feeling to give or receive? Open your heart to receive more and have more gratitude.

I am sure the first two words I was taught as a child were "please" and "thank you" - they are still the most important words for me to remember. I am pleased you have taken the time to read these messages and thank you for sharing.

I am in gratitude for all life. All is in Divine Right Order.

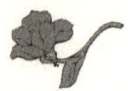

MESSAGE TWENTY-TWO

SEPARATION

We have never been separated from source but we have often forgotten how connected we truly are. In our dark moments of the soul we have been able to surrender to ourselves in compassion and humility, understanding how to find peace within our Being-ness. Going within is part of the balance for our busy lives. I believe praying (often in desperation or as a last resort!) is sending out a message to the god-force for help, guidance and support. Meditation is a measure of patience to receive the answers.

Living on the earth plane is like a school of work and play is our time out. I believe that when life is all work and no play it is time to re-evaluate to ensure balance and equanimity for the benefit of our well being. We are human creatures of habit – 'tis best to let go of the old habits, whose "use-by-date" is up and introduce a better habit. Opportunities are on our path always to make the changes necessary for our soul's growth – awareness is the key. Openness and honesty with others and ourselves are essential. How do we become more open and honest when our fears have limited our energies? By allowing ourselves to be vulnerable to life, people and circumstances. This is an act of humility; however discretion and discernment are needed otherwise if the pendulum of balance swings too far vulnerability becomes stupidity!

To value ourselves as a unique spark of energy is to keep our equilibrium – this is self-love and recognition of our spiritual mission, which assures us All is in Divine Right Order. We are here for the experience of understanding ourselves and giving service on the planet as a catalyst for change. We are spiritually guided and supported by the Universe. Remember that and you will not forget that you have come from source, are connected to source, are the essence of source and return to source.

The intuitive make-up of our psyche loves to play and the more lightness and brightness we allow in our lives, the more synchronicity we can manifest with others. Often one needs to laugh at and honour one's own idiosyncrasies to maintain the balance of light and dark. To find peace within is to find the sacred spaces and times to value oneself – otherwise life might not be worth the living.

A difficult life asks the question "how do I make my life easier?" By thinking and acting lighter we will attract brighter situations, as we will be able to recognise that out of every adversity come the seeds of greater benefits. Patience and compassion with self bring about humility that is understanding. Judge not until you fully understand and when you fully understand judgement is not necessary!

To SURRENDER is to TRUST that all is in Divine Right Order but often, due to our insecurities (which are a lack of love) we are afraid to surrender. The ego personality wants to protect us and we find we are reacting to our situations instead of responding. To be in a strong balanced state of being is to have peace within, self-love to then be able to respond with your own passion for life and consequently attract pros-perity.

Peace, passion and prosperity are the ultimate power of life on the earth plane. Power is energy used positively for balance, equilibrium of All-That-Is. Those of us who are seers – see into the future and with this picture are able to think this process into manifestation. We are all capable of becoming seers – it is just one's intuitive instinct enhanced and energised to a positive fullness of psychic empowerment.

To rest, relax and rejuvenate enables one's physical body (the temple) to harmonise with its mind (the will) and the soul (the god-force).

I AM ALL THAT I AM!

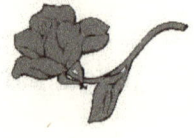

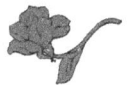

MESSAGE TWENTY-THREE

SENSITIVITY

Some people seem to be more sensitive with themselves, other people and the environment than others are. Also, some people will acknowledge that they become more sensitive to themselves, others and their environment as they become more aware of life's frailties and strengths.

The children of today seem to be more sensitive than the children of my day, however this is only our awareness being more perceptive these days. In actual fact, our gauge of sensitivity is entirely of our own making, governed by our soul's mission and how we fulfil our life's purpose. All highly creative souls are very sensitive and many children here on planet Earth today are here to teach their parents and others to 'STOP, LOOK and LISTEN' to them. Children who are labelled ADD, ADHD and Schizophrenics are prime examples. Their soul's mission can indeed be a difficult one but is made easier when others around them try to understand them on a spiritual level.

My mother was an evolving old soul (in numerology terms) and I was born the old soul into the family – she was frustrated by her sensitive, over exuberant child who was also the second born. Part of Mother's soul's mission was to learn from me and thus become more sensitive and understanding of herself. Mother died of cancer, carrying within her much resentment and guilt but her creative abilities were many and she left behind a beautiful home and garden which was her legacy for us all – foundations that are often necessary in this life.

When my mother came to me from the spirit world many years later she told me that she wanted to return to the earth plane to experience more of life's opportunities that she had not managed well previously and that she would need to return as a more sensitive soul to do so. I jokingly replied "Well, please don't come too near me for those experiences!" She replied that she needed to come as the first child in the next generation, as that is the way Karmic patterns are worked through and out. I know this to be true and was curious at the time as none of my children were intending to have a baby, but two and a half years later this miraculous event took place. Her spirit chose a family with lovely homes and gardens as foundations. As a highly sensitive being this child has many creative talents and has parents who Stop, Look, Listen and PLAY with him.

I recognise through this situation just how important "play" is in our lives, to allow our creative talents to manifest and have the confidence to follow through with them. In my period as a child there seemed to be an over-emphasis on discipline. Those of us with strict, limiting parents often in poverty consciousness, plus boarding school disciplines and limitations (usually religious) had the option of becoming rebellious! Although we seemed to be rebelling against the "systems", we were actually dynamic catalysts for the changes that are needed and continue to shape not only our own lives and soul's mission but others lives also.

To rebel is to be courageous and that can be lots of fun. All my careers or so-called professions have started from a hobby that was fun - living my passion. Even my marriage was a great adventure with three creative children as a result, and one of them was certainly a rebellious child. It was the number two child of course who now has three very sensitive children himself.

Part of our soul's mission is choosing our parents and the family circumstances which brings about our genetic coding as well - all to furnish ourselves as an evolving energy being having an adventure in consciousness on Mother Earth. The more we love and respect our foundations the easier our adventure can be - but remember when life becomes all work and no play the creative abilities will be limited and stifled. HAVE FUN - LIVE YOUR PASSION!

FOOTNOTE: There is a powerful message in the SERENITY POEM for all sensitives:

GRANT US THE SERENITY
TO ACCEPT THE THINGS WE CANNOT CHANGE
THE COURAGE TO CHANGE THE THINGS WE CAN
AND THE WISDOM TO KNOW THE DIFFERENCE

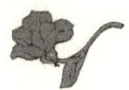

MESSAGE TWENTY-FOUR

THE UNIVERSE

The Universe is a Symbol of the God-force and we are the Co-creators. When I walked into my bathroom one evening and saw an incredible clear white symbol on the bathroom window, I asked, "What is the meaning of this?" The answer I received was WHOLENESS (from) SOURCE.

We are all WHOLENESS. This was a profound confirmation of what I had been coming to terms with in my life – that we are indeed whole and not apart from anything in the Universe. To reach this understanding I suggest you focus on the soul's purpose as a priority, understanding self, and then the mind becomes the director, the will, and your body the vehicle, the temple.

To resonate with nature is to be in tune with the whole, as nature is whole, a reflection of light, colour and sound, of All-That-Is and we are a reflection of light, colour, sound and All-That-Is.

Know that we are whole, the total sum of all our parts we call the human being. Such a miraculous vehicle/temple we have that has an amazing technology within itself to heal and grow in consciousness. So clever in fact, that scientists are really only finding out what we already know. We are the tick-tock of the Universal clock and when operating on TRUST, our communications with each other propel the circulatory systems of our bodies. Have you recognised how much better the circulation of your blood is when you are open, honest and communicating with others in a sharing capacity?

Our Third Dimensional life is all about communication and circulation for business success. We are the co-creators of that empire of materialism, which only manifests for us to the extent of our spiritual purpose.

We are all intrinsically part of the great whole of everything and sometimes, when our lives change completely, to become more focussed on our inner balance (which is also the balance of the whole Universe) we will be able to say "Been There, Done That!" We have done our creative good in that area and move on to let others move in for their experience. Life is about being creatively involved to have the experiences that bring about wisdom.

To teach from the heart is to teach from experience and wisdom – to lead by example. I have found that every message I have ever given as a communication to students or clients has always asked of my own self to exemplify.

As horses have five times greater perception than the average human being I am able to glean from my experiences with them to fulfil my measure of wisdom more subtly and profoundly. Horses' intelligence comes from their third eye. ESP is the technology of the future that will surpass computers, which are only here now to act as a bridge to mankind's brain. As one develops total TRUST in one's own INTUITION - higher self, and utilises it accordingly, one values the synchronicity that life presents with our communications. To develop this INTUITIVE power is to also develop psychic power—ESP - Extra Sensory Perception. This is totally possible for all, as the ability is a natural part of our psyche. To be able to have a conscious awareness of our intuitive capabilities to enhance our everyday lives is the key to TRUST in our spiritual selves and therefore trust in the process of our lives. FEAR is the trap that will prevent this development.

Glean from little children - they are our mirrors of remembering what we have forgotten, due to our fear related experiences in this life and often past lives too. Take time out in your balance of life to be totally relaxed and have fun - that is the best scenario for your intuition to keep you on track with your soul's purpose and further your journey.

The intuition opens the right brain fully - the creative brain that sees the whole picture and THEN the left-brain can do the analysing and put the picture into action. All nature is a reflection of our natural balance. All nature is a reflection of All-That-Is-LIGHT, LOVE, COLOUR and SOUND. Your SOUL, MIND and BODY are the Symbol of the Universe. The Universe is but One Vast Symbol of the God-force.

FOCUS

I have become conscious to every breath I take
For my healing, my innate ability.
I have become conscious to every step I take
To stay on my path, to surrender and trust.

I have become conscious to every negative thought I have
To change them, 'cos energy follows thought.
I have become conscious to every positive thought I have
For transformation, we all want it.

I have become conscious to every feeling I have
To transmute them, feelings are experiential.
I have become conscious of my metaphysical body
To understand the purpose, of my spiritual journey.

I have become conscious of my soul's mission
To manifest my dreams & goals, as a catalyst for change.
I have become conscious of my work related actions
To discipline myself, for my material success.

I have become conscious of every word I say
To stay in my power, power is my magnificence.
I have become conscious of every deed I do
To be an example, humanity needs us all.

I have become conscious as an Energy being
I am God, Goddess anchoring, Heaven-on earth.
I have become conscious of All-That-Is
Because we're all connected, to make a difference.

I have become conscious of cosmic energy
To grow in Love and Light, in the Universal plan.
I have become conscious of the present, now moment
To feel the essence within, of Love personified.

THE AUTHOR

Rose-marie was the first registered Metaphysical and Spiritual Counselor in New Zealand in the 1990's. A Reiki Master, Holistic Teacher, Intuitive Healer for twenty years.

For fifteen years she used a form of Colour Therapy to support and heal over fifty horses at her Quarter Horse Stud.

Other modalities Rose-marie has since added include:

NLP and Hypnotherapy
TFT and Quantum Touch
Alchemist and Vibrational Essences
Numerologist and Author of four books.

Rose-marie believes there is a cure for everything, when one wants to be cured and finds the answers to the imbalances. An attitude of gratitude is essential.

www.ingramcontent.com/pod-product-compliance
Lightning Source LLC
Chambersburg PA
CBHW032010080426
42735CB00007B/559